The Life of Sophia Jex-Blake

Condensed Edition

Margaret Todd, M.D.

Contents

Publishing Information

- (c) 2024 Nimble Books LLC
- ISBN: 978-1-60888-340-0
- Nimble Books LLC ~ NimbleBooks.com
- Fred Zimmerman, Editor

Bibliographic Key Phrases

Sophia Jex-Blake; feminist movement; women in medicine; medical education for women; women's suffrage; feminist pioneers; female education; medical practice; the Woman Question; social reform; University of Edinburgh; The Royal Infirmary; The Royal Free Hospital; The London School of Medicine for Women; feminist struggles; Victorian era; women's rights; medical history; women's history.

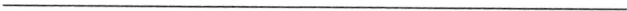

Publisher's Note

Are you looking for inspiration in a world often defined by relentless pressures and expectations? Do you crave a story that speaks to the enduring power of a single person to defy the odds and champion a cause bigger than themselves? Then *The Life of Sophia Jex-Blake* is a must-read. This captivating biography details the life of one of the most remarkable women of the 19th century, who dared to challenge a deeply entrenched societal order by fighting for the right of women to study medicine. Through a meticulous account of S. J.-B.'s life, from childhood through her struggles for a medical education and the founding of the first medical schools for women, author Margaret Todd reveals the raw, personal, and ultimately triumphant narrative of a pioneer breaking down barriers. This compelling story offers a unique look at the struggles women faced in the pursuit of higher education and professional opportunities. It underscores the power of an individual to be a force for positive change, particularly in a time when societal norms seemed set in stone. You'll discover how S. J.-B. navigated the complexities of Victorian society, faced fierce opposition, and ultimately transformed the landscape of medical education. With its vivid detail, insightful observations, and the personal insights found in S. J.-B.'s own diaries and letters, *The Life of Sophia Jex-Blake* is a must-read for anyone seeking inspiration and wanting to understand the remarkable efforts of those who paved the way for a more equitable world.

Truth in Publishing

This book, by Margaret Todd (Graham Travers), a Scottish physician, is a loving tribute to Sophia Jex-Blake, the first woman to obtain a medical degree in Great Britain. The story of Sophia Jex-Blake's life is engrossing, but the reader will have to navigate several challenges along the way.

Strengths:

- The text is an excellent example of a biography written by someone who knew and admired her subject. You'll learn a great deal about Sophia's life, and the book provides a fascinating window into the world of Victorian-era women and their fight for equal rights.
- The author's writing is elegant and detailed, though not all of her stylistic choices would be

considered "modern" today.

- The text is well-researched, providing a rich collection of letters and excerpts from the subject's diary.

Weaknesses:

- Be prepared for an onslaught of Victorian clichés—including the overuse of "darling" and "precious"—and some saccharine religious sentimentality. The author does her best to convey the zeitgeist, but her portrayal of the subject's spiritual life is often heavy-handed.
- At times, the author's tone descends into a tedious litany of reproaches. You'll be subjected to a relentless barrage of "S.J.-B. felt very unhappy" and "S.J.-B. felt very tired." And, despite the author's admirable admiration for her subject, the text is peppered with phrases that will make modern readers cringe, such as "How remarkable it is that a woman can have so much strength of character" or "How much this woman's character is due to her being *so* well-born."
- The author's tendency to excessive detail can be a drag. You'll discover more than you ever wanted to know about the subject's dress, dietary habits, and finances. Be warned: This book is a "Sinker" if you're not ready for a deep dive.

Overall:

In the end, this is a good read that gives a compelling picture of a remarkable woman. But be prepared to wade through an overabundance of clichés and some frustratingly repetitive language to get there. If you're looking for a light and breezy read, this is not it. But if you are interested in a deeply personal, well-researched exploration of the life of a courageous and intelligent woman, then this might be just what you are looking for.

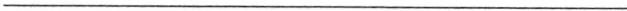

Historical Context

Margaret Georgina Todd's *The Life of Sophia Jex-Blake* was published in 1918, a tumultuous year in which the first World War ended and the Spanish flu ravaged the globe. The social landscape was equally in flux as the Victorian era gave way to a more modern era of individualism and social reform. This biography appeared in the midst of a nascent but powerful feminist movement. The fight for women's suffrage was in full swing, and women were also agitating for expanded education and employment opportunities, a theme that is central to *The Life of Sophia Jex-Blake*. The book's publication coincided with the growth of The National Association for the Education of Women in 1916, a US group dedicated to promoting the medical education of women. Its publication helped to galvanize public sentiment in support of the women's medical education movement.

The 1867 *Reform Act* had granted the vote to working-class men in Great Britain, but not to women. The publication of John Stuart Mill's *The Subjection of Women* in 1869 further spurred debate on the rights of women. While Jex-Blake's fight for women's access to medical education began in the 1860s, her campaign achieved a higher profile after the *Reform Act* of 1867, as did similar struggles for women's rights in education and professions in general.

While women's suffrage became a key topic in the late 19th century and the early 20th century, the movement for women's access to medical education also grew, particularly in the wake of Jex-Blake's efforts.

Her efforts, and the resulting biography, became a powerful symbol of the fight for women's rights and equality. *The Life of Sophia Jex-Blake* contributed to the expanding discourse on women's rights and challenged the traditional role of women in society. In subsequent years, the book continued to be an important document in the feminist movement.

The Life of Sophia Jex-Blake remains relevant today, given the continued fight for women's rights and the increasing prominence of women in professional and leadership roles. This book provides a historical and personal perspective on the challenges faced by women in the Victorian era, and their struggles to overcome these in a social context where women were still confined to a narrow range of options in education, work, and family life.

The book also provides historical context to the continued debate about gender equality, particularly in the medical field, with more than one reviewer taking pains to note the persistence of certain views expressed in the text, and its echoes in current, ongoing trends.

In 2018, #MeToo sparked a global movement of women (and some men) who voiced their opposition to sexual harassment, sexual assault, and sexual violence, a situation that echoes in the book's narrative of the women's battle with the male-dominated medical establishment, and with the more aggressive elements of the male student body.

A 2022 report from the World Health Organization on the State of the World's Midwifery, emphasizes the need to "strengthen the health workforce and invest in the education, training and employment of more midwives." In several respects, the report and its recommendations stand testament to Jex-Blake's achievement, given her early, passionate advocacy in the realm of women's healthcare and the challenges she faced.

The Life of Sophia Jex-Blake is a reminder that the battle for women's equality in all areas of human endeavor is a slow and continuous struggle, with a history far longer than the events of the late 19th and early 20th centuries that are documented in the text. In the coming decades, it is likely that the work will continue to be an important resource for feminist historians, and for anyone interested in the evolution of the women's movement for social and professional equality.

Abstracts

TLDR (three words)

Woman fights for medicine.

ELI5

This is a story about a brave girl named Sophia who wanted to be a doctor. It was really hard for girls to become doctors in the old days, so Sophia had to fight for her dream. She went to school, went to college, and then went to medical school, but people kept trying to stop her. She was really smart and brave, and in the end, she became a doctor, and many other women followed in her footsteps.

Scientific-Style Abstract

This biography of Sophia Jex-Blake charts her struggles to obtain medical education in England and Scotland. As a child and adolescent, Jex-Blake expressed her unique personality in a way that caused consternation to her family, a theme that continued throughout her life as she pushed against the constraints of Victorian society. Jex-Blake's experiences in the United States, her close friendship with Octavia Hill, and her battle to gain entry to Edinburgh University and to the Royal Infirmary are detailed, as is her subsequent success in obtaining medical degrees in Switzerland and Ireland. This account of a woman who fought for her right to a profession will be of interest to historians and to all those who have a regard for the pursuit of equality.

For Complete Idiots Only

This book is about a woman named Sophia Jex-Blake who was a complete pain in the neck to everyone but fought to become a doctor.

Learning Aids

Mnemonic (acronym)

S.J.-B. stood for:

- **S**tudent - She was the first woman to matriculate in the University of Edinburgh.
- **J**ournalist - She wrote articles and books on her experiences.
- **B**attle - She fought against sexism and social prejudice in the medical field.

Mnemonic (speakable)

Sophy's life was a story of *Sackermena and her Isles*, a world she created as a child, **Queen's College**, where she excelled, but was frustrated by the rigid, Victorian atmosphere. She went to **Germany**, but returned with renewed dedication and a desire to be a **Doctor**. She was met with resistance, but never gave up the **Fight**.

Mnemonic (singable)

(To the tune of "Oh, My Darling, Clementine")

> In Hastings, England, she was born, A little girl so full of scorn, She dreamed of an island, Sweet Sackermena, And a world of perfect laws was born.

> The rules of Victorian school, Sophy never would be ruled, She was a wild child, Sweet Sackermena, And in her heart she knew she would be cool.

> To London she went, Queen's College she spent With professors great, Sweet Sackermena, And the idea of medicine was sent.

> To Edinburgh she went, To open the university gate, A tough and long fight, Sweet Sackermena, To make medicine a woman's fate.

> To the Infirmary she went, A riot her presence would present, The "Irish Brigade"

Sweet Sackermena, For her protection
they would be sent.

She studied and fought, The battle was
long sought, She won a degree, Sweet
Sackermena, And made a woman doctor
free.

In Sussex she lived, A garden she thrived,
And loved her old friends, Sweet Sackermena, Till her life at last she did end.

Analytic Table of Contents

Part I

Chapter I: Childhood

This chapter discusses the birth and childhood of Sophia Jex-Blake, with an emphasis on her close relationship with her parents and the influence of their deeply religious upbringing. We are also introduced to her early artistic tendencies, particularly her creation of the imaginary kingdom of Sackermena and her Isles.

Chapter II: School Life

The author explores S. J.-B.'s stormy, often unhappy,

school years, where she is frequently chastised for her outspokenness, lack of conventional femininity and, above all, her tendency to "make people uncomfortable." She struggles to conform to the standards of piety expected of her and is labelled a "terrible pickle" by her teachers and classmates.

Chapter III: School Life—Continued

S. J.-B.'s school days continue to be marked by challenges, including poor physical health that is misinterpreted and treated as a sign of a troubled mind. While her innate intelligence is evident, S. J.-B. fails to meet expectations, in part due to the restrictive nature of girls' education at the time.

Chapter IV: School Life—Concluded

This chapter marks the end of S. J.-B.'s formal schooling, where she is expelled for her disobedience and lack of "ladylike" behavior. She is entrusted to the care of her former schoolmistress, Mrs. Teed, where she undergoes a period of religious introspection. A letter from her father on the plight of the Crimean soldiers sheds light on the social and political issues of the time. S. J.-B.'s heartfelt letter to her father expressing her own doubts and fears about her religious life and behavior sheds light on her early development.

Chapter V: Life at Home

This chapter examines S. J.-B.'s life at home after leaving school, where she continues to struggle with her parents over expectations of conforming to societal norms. She harbors dreams of becoming an author and grapples with feelings of self-absorption and depression. A pivotal moment comes when she is introduced to two Norfolk cousins, Elinor and Sarah Jex-Blake, who help to transform her outlook on life.

Chapter VI: Life at Queen's College

The author follows S. J.-B. as she enters Queen's College in 1858, a new institution of higher learning for women, where she encounters friction and difficulties in finding suitable lodgings. She is appointed mathematical tutor and engages in a spirited correspondence with her father concerning accepting payment for her work. She successfully completes her course and is awarded a certificate "with great credit."

Chapter VII: Friendship

This chapter discusses S. J.-B.'s multifaceted personality and her capacity for friendship. We are introduced to her friendship with Miss Octavia Hill, who begins as a teacher and becomes a close confidante, providing both comfort and a challenge to her.

Chapter VIII: A Step Beyond

This chapter discusses the significant impact of her

friendship with Octavia Hill on S. J.-B. It is a turning point in her life, marking a time of self-reflection and a greater commitment to her religious faith, a faith she describes as a "grand solemn wonder," freeing her from the burden of personal pain.

Chapter IX: First Experience of Edinburgh

S. J.-B. travels to Edinburgh seeking advanced education, but is disappointed with the quality of instruction available to women. She embarks on a varied course of study, engages with the city's religious and political life and is supported by a small circle of close friends. She discusses her ongoing theological struggles with her mother and consults with Rev. Dr. Pulsford, who provides some guidance, but ultimately encourages her to "live it out."

Chapter X: Germany

The author discusses S. J.-B.'s decision to continue her studies abroad, with a focus on her time spent in Germany. We learn about her efforts to obtain medical education, her initial disappointment with the quality of instruction, her decision to seek teaching opportunities and her eventual appointment as an English teacher at the Grand Ducal Institute in Mannheim.

Chapter XI: Life as a Teacher at Mannheim

This chapter depicts S. J.-B.'s life as an English teacher in Mannheim, where she is confronted with cultural differences and a strict "no holiday" system. Her letters to her mother provide a glimpse into her experiences and her changing views on religious dogma.

Chapter XII: Various Projects and Ventures

The author describes S. J.-B.'s time back home in England after her stay in Mannheim. She experiences a period of ill-health and considers various ventures, including becoming a Lady Principal of a girls' school in Manchester. This chapter also includes her visit to America where she further explores the education of women and begins her own journey towards a medical career.

Chapter XIII: A Visit to Some American Schools and Colleges

This chapter traces S. J.-B.'s visit to the United States, where she observes American educational practices and is deeply impressed by the co-education of men and women in the colleges she visits. Her observations lead her to compare American and English education. We also learn about her first encounters with women doctors and her growing interest in a medical career.

Chapter XIV: Questionings

This chapter describes S. J.-B.'s experience as a dispenser and volunteer at the New England Hospital for Women, where she becomes increasingly drawn to the field of medicine. Her internal struggles over her calling in life and her evolving religious beliefs are highlighted.

Chapter XV: Pioneer Work in America

S. J.-B.'s decision to pursue a medical career is marked by a series of efforts to gain admission to Harvard Medical School. She is ultimately rejected, but finds opportunities for clinical teaching at Massachusetts General Hospital and private anatomy lessons in New York.

Chapter XVI: Going Home

This chapter recounts S. J.-B.'s return to England, her continued interest in medical study, her father's illness and subsequent death. Her mother's constant support is emphasized, as is the growing distance between S. J.-B. and her brother, who still has difficulty understanding her.

Part II

Chapter I: Drifting

S. J.-B. returns to Brighton after her father's death and contemplates her future. She is torn between her desire to pursue a medical career and her commitment to her mother.

Chapter II: At the Gates of the Citadel

This chapter delves into S. J.-B.'s decision to pursue her medical studies, which leads her to Edinburgh, where she seeks to gain admission to the prestigious Edinburgh University. She begins canvassing professors and other influential individuals, seeking support for her application.

Chapter III: Success?

The author highlights S. J.-B.'s efforts to gain the approval of the Medical Faculty, who, after much deliberation, decide in her favor. She is then granted tentative permission to study at the university. The support of the *Scotsman*, a leading newspaper, is a significant factor in this success.

Chapter IV: A Check

Despite initial successes, S. J.-B. encounters opposition. Professor Christison, a prominent figure in the medical community, opposes her application. The University Court, a higher authority, overturns the Senatus's decision, preventing her from continuing her studies.

Chapter V: Opening of Edinburgh University to Women

This chapter describes the renewed efforts of S. J.-B. and other women in supporting the cause of women's medical education in Edinburgh. The author highlights the role of Mrs. Thorne and Miss Pechey in this campaign. She also discusses the efforts of Dr. King Chambers to secure admission for women at St. Mary's Hospital, which ultimately fail. However, the University Court agrees to admit women to separate classes.

Chapter VI: The Hope Scholarship

The author discusses the difficulties faced by S. J.-B. and her fellow students in finding qualified teachers, and how the university fails to award the Hope Scholarship to Edith Pechey, despite her success in the examination.

Chapter VII: Practical Difficulties

The author focuses on the difficulties faced by the women in securing adequate teaching and examination, particularly in the field of anatomy.

Chapter VIII: The Riot at Surgeons' Hall

This chapter details a crucial turning point in the fight for women's medical education in Edinburgh. S. J.-B. and her fellow students are prevented from entering Surgeons' Hall and are subjected to a riot, where they are shouted at, jeered, and even pelted with mud.

Chapter IX: The Action for Libel

Professor Christison's assistant files a libel lawsuit against S. J.-B. for her statements concerning his behavior during the riot. S. J.-B. is supported by her brother and friends and makes an impassioned speech at a suffrage meeting in London.

Chapter X: Some Friendships and Holidays

The author highlights the support S. J.-B. received from various individuals, including a public subscription to defray the costs of the lawsuit. She also discusses her holiday in Paris, where she witnesses the effects of the Commune.

Chapter XI: The Question of Professional Examination

The women face continued obstacles in gaining access to adequate teaching and examination. They are refused entry into the first professional examination but are admitted and pass after a letter is sent to the examiners by their lawyer.

Chapter XII: The Royal Infirmary

The author discusses the ongoing struggle of the women students to continue their medical education in Edinburgh. She emphasizes the support they received from various individuals, including Professor Sidgwick and Mr. James Stuart. The women's party at the Infirmary's annual meeting results in a victory that allows them to be admitted to separate classes.

Chapter XIII: The Action Against the Senatus

The author recounts the legal battle between S. J.-B. and other women students against the Senatus of the University of Edinburgh. The aim is to clarify the women's status as students.

Chapter XIV: The Lord Ordinary's Judgment

This chapter describes S. J.-B.'s lecture in London on the medical education of women. She highlights the differences of opinion between herself and Mrs. Butler. S. J.-B. publishes *Medical Women*, a book about the historical fight for women's medical education. Lord Ordinary makes a decision substantially in favor of the women students.

Chapter XV: Paying the Price

S. J.-B. is rejected from the first professional examination, leading to newspaper coverage and public support. She is criticized for her failure and the University appeals the Lord Ordinary's decision.

Chapter XVI: End of the Battle in Edinburgh

The women students continue their studies despite the University's continued opposition. S. J.-B. engages in politics and helps to elect women to the Edinburgh

School Board. The University appeals the Lord Ordinary's decision, but the Court of Session decides by a narrow majority in favor of the University. The women are encouraged to pursue their education at other institutions in Britain and Ireland.

Chapter XVII: The Question in Parliament

This chapter explores the increasing public and newspaper interest in the plight of the women students. Mrs. Anderson writes a letter to the *Times* advising women to study abroad and practice without registration, to which S. J.-B. responds. A bill is introduced in Parliament to remove the legal obstacles to the medical education of women in Scotland. The bill fails to pass, but the debate brings the question into the realm of practical politics.

Chapter XVIII: The London School of Medicine for Women

The author recounts the founding of the London School of Medicine for Women, which was prompted by S. J.-B.'s rejection from the Edinburgh examinations, the ongoing parliamentary debate and the persistent discrimination faced by women in the medical field.

Chapter XIX: The Russell Gurney Enabling Act

S. J.-B. and her colleagues are unsuccessful in securing

the passage of two separate bills, but the Government finally indicates its willingness to support a "Foreign Degrees Bill," which is then passed. The Irish College of Surgeons is prompted to open its examinations to women, leading to a greater sense of hope.

Chapter XX: At Last

This chapter details how S. J.-B. and Miss Pechey, unable to secure a medical degree in England, complete their studies at the University of Berne and achieve their long-sought goal of obtaining the Licentiate of the Irish College.

Chapter XXI: The Royal Free Hospital

The author discusses the efforts of S. J.-B. and her colleagues to gain admission for women students to the Royal Free Hospital, which is eventually granted. This victory marks a turning point for women in medicine in London and the entire United Kingdom. We also learn about the opening of London University to women and S. J.-B.'s role in the organization of the London School for Women.

Part III

Chapter I: Early Days in Practice

The author details S. J.-B.'s early years of practice in Edinburgh. She describes the initial difficulties faced by women doctors, particularly S. J.-B. as the first woman doctor in Scotland. She also discusses S. J.-B.'s unique approach to patient care and her commitment to social justice.

Chapter II: Last Illness of Mrs. Jex-Blake

This chapter describes the final illness and death of S. J.-B.'s mother. It highlights the close and loving relationship between mother and daughter and S. J.-B.'s selfless devotion to her mother's care.

Chapter III: Patients and Friends

The author follows S. J.-B. after her mother's death as she moves to Bruntsfield Lodge and establishes a new life and practice in Edinburgh. She discusses her deep and lasting friendships with the women who supported her throughout her career, including Miss Du Pre.

Chapter IV: Public Life

The author discusses S. J.-B.'s continued involvement in public life, including her work in support of women's rights, her writings on social issues, and her involvement in efforts to secure a charter for the Edinburgh Extra-Mural School.

Chapter V: Re-Opening of Edinburgh University to Women

This chapter highlights the culmination of the fight for the medical education of women in Edinburgh. The University of Edinburgh finally opens its doors to women after a struggle that spanned over twenty-five years. The author discusses S. J.-B.'s contributions to this historic victory, her work as a lecturer in midwifery and her continued commitment to supporting her students.

Chapter VI: Driving Tours. Animal Friends

The author examines S. J.-B.'s love of the outdoors and her deep connection to animals. She describes her passion for driving tours, her relationship with her horses and her special affection for her cat, Karma.

Chapter VII: The Sabbatical Year

This chapter recounts S. J.-B.'s decision to retire and the events that led to her search for a suitable home in Sussex. Her decision to purchase Windydene, where she enjoys a life of seclusion, gardening, and hospitality. The author also discusses her enduring friendships and her continuing interest in public affairs.

Appendix A: Pedigree of the Jex-Blake Family. Origin of compound surname

This appendix traces the lineage of the Jex-Blake family, providing historical context for the origin of their surname.

Appendix B: "Words for the Way"—No. 2. Rest

This appendix presents one of S. J.-B.'s three tracts written to address religious topics in a non-doctrinal way.

Appendix C: Conclusions from "A Visit to American Schools and Colleges"

This appendix offers excerpts from S. J.-B.'s book, *A Visit to Some American Schools and Colleges*, highlighting her observations of American education and her views on co-education.

Appendix D: The Edinburgh Extra-Mural School

This appendix provides information about the Edinburgh Extra-Mural School and its relationship with the University of Edinburgh.

Appendix E: Letter to the *Times* in reply to Mrs. Garrett Anderson

This appendix includes S. J.-B.'s response to Mrs. Garrett Anderson's letter to the *Times*, in which she argues against Mrs. Anderson's suggestion that women should seek medical education abroad.

Appendix F: Letter to the *Times* in reply to the Principal of Edinburgh University

This appendix includes a letter to the *Times* from the Principal of Edinburgh University that defends the University's actions. S. J.-B.'s response to the letter corrects factual inaccuracies and reiterates her view that the University had unjustly obstructed the women students.

Appendix G: Permanent Memorials of S. J.-B.

This appendix details the memorials in honor of S. J.-B.'s life and work that are located at St. Giles' Cathedral, Edinburgh, the Edinburgh Hospital for Women and Children, the family monument at Ovingdean, and Rotherfield Churchyard.

Condensed Matter

The Condensed Matter section begins with Sophia Jex-Blake's childhood and education. She was precocious, but rebellious. Here's her story.

Sophia was born in 1840 to loving and devoted parents:

> "How happy I was with my Baby this time two and twenty years ago!" writes Mrs. Jex-Blake on the 21st January, 1862, and, if she had greater cause than some mothers for the plaintive note that one seems to hear through the words, she was the first to rejoice in her great compensations.

> Certainly no baby ever had a warmer welcome into the world.

Her parents were Evangelicals, but also aristocrats:

> What made this attitude all the finer was
> the fact that neither husband nor wife was
> ever tempted to undervalue social distinc-
> tions. It was *noblesse oblige* always,—the
> *noblesse* of family as much as the *noblesse*
> of Christ.

Young Sophia was a bit of a handful:

> And, for better or worse, into this at-
> mosphere Sophia Jex-Blake was born.
> One can scarcely wonder that she came
> as a little queen. "Brother" was already
> at school, his foot on the first step of a
> brilliant career; "Sweet Carrie" was all that
> loving parents expected her to be; the new
> thing came as a complete surprise. The
> freshness, the wilfulness, the naughtiness
> of her were as the wine of life to these
> staid, law-abiding people. It took their
> breath away sometimes, but it was all
> on so small a scale, and were not all the
> forces of religion in reserve to check any
> undue waywardness as soon as she was old
> enough to understand?

One of her early educational experiences was an exten-
sive family tour of the Lake District:

They visited Leamington, Warwick, Kenilworth: thence to Edinburgh, Stirling, Glasgow and the Lochs, Callander and the Trossachs, stopping at York on the way south.

She went to a series of schools, and wasn't a model student:

If we bear in mind what the state of girls' education was in those days we shall see that it could scarcely have been otherwise. If she could have gone to a boys' school and enjoyed its boisterous give and take, the little "despotic emperor" would soon have found her level. One loves to think how happy she would have been in the modern Girls' High School: if she had but found the education of women in the condition in which she left it, the difference in her whole future would have been very great, but women of the present day would not owe her the debt they owe her now. "The breaker is gone up before them."

She chafed under the rules and restrictions:

"I *exceedingly* like a letter from you, and bustle down a little earlier on Tuesday morning that I may have time to enjoy it before breakfast.... Cousins Kate and Elinor Jex-Blake say they do not at all delight in Mathematics, they are sorry to say."

"We are very sorry to disappoint you, but indeed we cannot sanction your going to see the 'Wizard of the North.' I do hope and believe you will submit cheerfully to give up what it would make me very sleepless and unhappy to have you go to. Now get a victory and believe the disappointment all for the best."

"Though I am most decidedly better, it arises, I think, from *perfect quiet*, the least change or bustle brings on spasm or headache, or both. Carry had Punch, and thought you sent it. I don't like it, I think it a vulgar paper, and don't wish it sent. I don't at all object to the 'Illustrated News' occasionally."

She was an exceptional student:

One has to remind oneself constantly— what the daughter never forgot, though small trace of it appears in the letters of this period—that Mrs. Jex-Blake had a keen sense of humour. When she and

Sophy were together, they had many a good joke in common. It was when the mesmerism of the child's presence was removed that the sense of responsibility asserted itself in full force. It is impossible to read the long series of letters without being profoundly convinced,—1. That the parents were devotedly attached to their youngest child ("Sophy was the favourite," was the elder sister's deliberate comment some sixty years later). 2. That their affection was returned with an intensity of which few children are capable. 3. That the warning that she was injuring her Mother's health and must therefore be kept away from her dearly-loved home did not provide a motive strong enough to make the child run in harness like other people. The inference is that no motive would have been strong enough.

Did she ever really make an honest effort? One comes upon many impassioned scraps of prayer for grace to resist temptation. "Oh, that when a word irritates me I may remember how often I have said more unkind things and been forgiven." "Oh, Lord, punish me, reduce me to submission in any way Thou seest fit, but oh, let me not alone,

abandon me not despite my wickedness."
And, although these prayers are apt to run
into conventional exaggerated language, it
is impossible to doubt their sincerity.

Her tiny booklets and papers were always
kept with the strictest secrecy, and it is all
but certain that no eye but her own ever
saw them before her death.

And she was very bright, as evidenced by the observations of her schoolmates, who were asked to write character sketches:

"Sophy is very affectionate and has more
good in her than people think, she is
truthful and can be trusted. She has an
immense amount of self-conceit, self-
sufficiency and pride. She will not be led
by anything but affection, or a desire to
make much of herself, and make herself
well thought of. She has great talents and
is very clever. She wishes to be thought an
out-of-the-way character and is so. She
lacks gentleness of feeling and manner."

Having finished school, Sophia Jex-Blake begins life at
home and then at Queen's College in London, but she
is restless and yearns to do more.

Sophia had great ambitions, but was also subject to

crippling self-doubt:

> Well, shall I be a great authoress as my day and night dreams prompt me to hope?... Shall I ever be a happy wife and mother? Shall I ere ten years, or half ten years have passed, be *dust*?... I sometimes think so. (June 1st. 1869. At any rate never thought of being a sawbones.)

She had a special relationship with her mother:

> And, Mother, about my marrying,—the chances pro and con. I said I did not fancy I should ever marry, for I thought I should require too many qualities to meet in the man I could think of as my husband, for it to be likely that I should ever meet such a paragon who could be willing to marry me.

Sophia became deeply involved in helping others less fortunate:

> I do not know when I could so fully and entirely say, 'I will lay me down *in peace* and sleep, for Thou, Lord, only makest me to dwell in safety.'"

In 1858, she started attending Queen's College:

> It is difficult for girl students of the present day to imagine all that was meant by

the opening of Queen's College in 1858. The plan of establishing a college for women had been much discussed by Alfred Tennyson, Charles Kingsley, and others; and the work had been warmly taken up by Frederick Denison Maurice, E. H. Plumptre (afterwards Dean of Wells) and R. C. Trench (afterwards Archbishop of Dublin), all three of whom were represented on the teaching staff. We may imagine what it meant for S. J.-B. to pass from the hands of the average schoolmistress of that day to teachers such as these.

She excelled in her studies:

She was "fay" that night, as they say in Scotland: it was scarcely lucky to be so happy. She little guessed, poor child, "what it would be to look back upon" her life at Queen's. Much happiness she got from that life, no doubt,—a rich harvest of education, contact with interesting temperaments and able minds, friendships that were only broken by death.

On the 5th October she settled down to work, and three days later she writes:

"Very delicious it is to be here. 'Oh, if there be an Elysium on earth, it is this, it is this!' I am inclined to say. I am as happy as a queen. Work and independence! What can be more charming? Really perfection. So delicious in the present, what will it be to look back upon?"

She was appointed mathematical tutor:

She had not been two months at College when she was asked to take the post of mathematical tutor. The suggestion gave her great pleasure, and she broached the subject to her parents when she next went home. Though startled, they were on the whole pleased at the honour done her, but things assumed a different aspect when her father realized the conditions on which the tutorship was to be held.

She had a serious falling-out with her father regarding the propriety of a lady accepting payment for her labor:

The correspondence seems well worth quoting *in extenso*:

This falling-out was quite painful for both, as they loved each other deeply. The debate continued for many letters. Sophia prevailed, and began to accept payment for tutoring.

So closes this delightful correspondence. It was not to be supposed that she should have no regrets. In her diary she says:

"Feb. 13th.... Like a fool I have consented to give up the fees for this term only—though I am miserably poor. I am sorry. It was foolish. It only defers the struggle."

Jex-Blake was a complex personality:

Elinor was the first to pay a visit to the unknown world, and she writes a long account of it to the eager Sarah:

"When I first saw her that evening, I thought she did not look so well, but since then I think the contrary—She is much thinner, but in good spirits, and so happy. I think she quite likes everyone to know that she has been made mathematical tutor, for it is considered a great honour."

S. J.-B. would fain have seen more of these delightful cousins, but their father held strict views as to the conditions under which well-born girls might visit London.

"You have taken yourself out of your natural position, and you cannot understand the need for their conforming to the proprieties their Father so naturally and properly expects. Good-looking girls do not needlessly go about London without chaperons. Happily for them, their Father's wish is sufficient to guide them. There is a respect and duty to the position, however weak and inferior you may judge a Parent to be. Well, darling, God bless and comfort you."

Yet, judged by present-day standards, S. J.-B. would not have been considered deficient in the spirit of compromise. Her letters to her Father on the subject of tutor's fees is evidence enough on that score, and those letters are in no way at variance with her whole attitude.

"A triumph as to *life*!" she records in her diary. "Last Monday told Mummy of my not going to the Opera without telling her, but proclaimed my intention in the future. No interdiction.

She continued her quest for more education and experience:

In any case S. J.-B. went straight on her course, like many of the finest girls of our own day, without giving any thought to cross currents that might alter the course of her life. And indeed her daily life was absorbing enough. It is scarcely surprising if, among her many interests, her religious life was somewhat smothered for the time, or that, at least she thought so.

She continued to be frustrated by the limitations of the available education for women:

On the last night of the year she writes:

"In this year my idea of work in the cause of education has developed itself into that of a resident College of the Holy Trinity. Heaven knows if ever to be carried out. If good,—yes, doubtless,—if not, God will raise up better. Little 'religious' as I fear I am, I do feel this thoroughly....

'And may the New Year cheri⧵
All the hopes that now are ⧵

Such a happy loving Goodnight to and from Daddy and Mummy. Very happy I am tonight.

'And once more ere thou per⧵
Old Year, Good night! Good ⧵

Sophia Jex-Blake begins to find herself. In this section, she experiences a transformative friendship with Octavia Hill and begins her battle for women's medical education in Edinburgh.

Jex-Blake was a young woman with a strong personality and, by this time, a strong sense of herself:

> In many ways she was developing; she was beginning, too, to take her full share of responsibility as regards her fellow-creatures, entering into the meaning of brotherhood and citizenship. In addition to her work at Queen's College, she undertook to teach bookkeeping gratuitously in connection with the Society for the Employment of Women, and had a class of children at Great Ormond Street. "I don't know how I should like *her*," said a candid critic, "but it is a pleasure to see anyone do anything so well as she does teach."

She was also highly capable of close, supportive friendships:

> If friendships are to be weighed, not counted, S. J.-B. was, even at this period, fortunate in her possession of them. The Norfolk cousins, the Cordery family, Miss Wodehouse, Miss Ada Benson, Miss Lucy Walker (afterwards Mrs. Unwin) who was her junior at Queen's, Miss Martha Heaton (Mrs. Hilhouse) a fellow teacher,—are the

names that occur to one most readily.

In 1860, she met Octavia Hill, and this friendship had a profound influence on her:

> And at this time there came into her life a friendship that was destined to make a deeper impression on her than any of these,—the deepest impression, in fact, of any in the whole of her life.

This is how it began:

> "Jan. 26th. 1860. Just had a lesson in book-keeping from Miss [Octavia] Hill. Clever, pleasant girl,—much nicer than I thought. Dined with me. What and how the deuce am I to pay her? £1 1s., I suppose. Dear old Patty Heaton! How fond I am of her, and what wonderfully good friends we are!"

> "Jan. 27th. I am sure I am a good companion for her (Miss Heaton) if only in amusing her. I think laughing does her a deal of good—hearty fun. I rejoice in her exceedingly. And I hope for another sort of friend, or ally at least, in Miss Hill who came and taught me book-keeping yesterday evening. Nice, sensible, clever. Very good worker, I expect."

They became very close:

> Almost from the first Miss Hill's letters to
> S. J.-B. took a serious tone. On March 18th
> she writes:

> "I wonder whether you will think me very
> impertinent if I say that I wonder you don't
> see that, in turning away from so many im-
> portant thoughts with a half joke, you are
> refusing God's means of grace as much as
> in staying away from ordained services. It
> is no good my writing sermons, however....
> I trust to live to see some one or some sor-
> row do for you what I cannot, to see such a
> peace as 'passeth all understanding' come
> over you, to see the thankful, perfect dedi-
> cation of all your powers to His service for
> His sake....

> I too long for a nice quiet talk with you. I
> enjoy it so, and your magnificent energy
> does me such good."

They decided to live together:

> It is therefore with no small sinking of
> heart that one reads the following entry in
> S. J.-B.'s diary:

> "Sept. 9th. Sunday [1860]. A plan on foot

of my taking part of a house with the Hills and having Alice for a servant. That would be very jolly. But rents high about here,—least £120."

Certainly a similar sinking of heart took possession of Mr. and Mrs. Jex-Blake, and when they learned that the finding of a tenant for the drawing-room floor was an essential part of the scheme, it is not surprising that—short of stopping their daughter's allowance which had been increased some time before—they did everything in their power to discourage the arrangement. They were well aware that, here as everywhere, the willing shoulders would take their full share of work and responsibility.

Ultimately, the arrangement didn't work, and Octavia moved out. The experience was deeply painful for Sophia:

"Bankrupt?" she asks herself. "No, by God's grace, no! No personal trouble, no trouble of any kind, *can* wreck a life in His charge. Still His,—that the strong, the enduring thought.

Eventually, she recovered from this setback and

resolved to go to Scotland to seek further education:

> "My life in Scotland to begin whenever rested."

She was disappointed in the available educational opportunities there. She also met and befriended Elizabeth Garrett:

> It was clear that there was nothing to be gained here, so next morning she "explained and apologised" to the Principal, and found him "very nice and pleasant." Her first impulse was to go straight back to London (in fact arrangements were made for her to live with Miss Wodehouse and study at Bedford College) but in the end wiser counsels prevailed.

> It is interesting to hear what she herself has to say about the various elements in her life referred to above:

> "There never was such a book as *Jane Eyre*—of its kind. Talk of 'finding'—that finds me through and through continually. How people *dare* speak ill of such a book,— I suppose they simply can't understand it. Its grand steadfastness and earnestness and purity, is something glorious. I read and re-read it as I never could another

novel, and how it helps one!"

"*Aids to Faith* put into my trunk by that dear old Mother who in her weaker moment entertains an uncomfortable kind of desire to proselytize me,—and yet can't be quite dissatisfied.

Immensely interested in *Aids to Faith*. Read Cook's Ideology and Subscription, Brown's 'Inspiration,' and am reading Mansel's 'Miracles.' The last gives me a glimpse of light and clearness I never had before.

It is clear that there was about her a doggedness, a high-handedness, a disregard of tradition, an actual—if superficial—roughness, which are not common qualities among the highly-educated of either sex, and which were never admired in her own.

On the other hand, the reader of the foregoing pages will no longer need to be told of her tenderness and sensitiveness—of a capacity for loving and for suffering only commensurate with her power of inspiring love, of incurring suffering.

She was coming into her own as an independent

woman:

In any case these first months in Edinburgh though she talks afterwards of their "grey pain," were perhaps the high-water mark of S. J.-B.'s life as regards sheer balance and beauty of living. She was having, it is true, no physical recreation, but, apart from that, her faculties were all called equally into play. She was working steadily and hard, chiefly at her beloved mathematics: her wider reading included *Jane Eyre*, *Le Juif Errant* and *Aids to Faith*: she was profoundly interested in religious problems and conscientiously attended the churches of the best-known Edinburgh ministers: she was happy in her friendships, and still more in the passing beauty of her relation to her Mother: above all, the flame of her religious life—in which was almost merged at this time her devotion to Miss Octavia Hill—was burning with a clearness that made it easy to ignore the little jars and frictions. Even politics were not crowded out. "Daddy is here," says Mrs. Jex-Blake in one of her letters, "and says, 'Tell dearest Sophy I would not have the *Times*, which she makes such excellent use of, given up on any account.' "

Having been rebuffed in her attempt to get a medical education at Edinburgh University, Sophia Jex-Blake moves to the United States, studies medicine, and, eventually, returns to Britain and opens a medical school in London.

Jex-Blake was a tireless advocate for women's education:

> The reader will recall, too, the letter to her Mother:

> "I am beginning to have hope, Mother! If I only suffer enough,—and I don't believe mine will ever be a smooth or easy life,—I may yet some day be fit to *be* the head for which I am looking so earnestly."

In the early 1860s, Elizabeth Garrett (later Anderson) had determined to become a doctor, and Jex-Blake befriended her:

> It was perhaps well that an interesting new factor came into S. J.-B.'s life at this moment. Miss Elizabeth Garrett (afterwards Mrs. Garrett Anderson, M.D.) had made up her mind to be a doctor, and, in the teeth of many difficulties and much opposition, was striving to obtain the requisite

education and prospect of examination.

Jex-Blake assisted Elizabeth in attempting to gain admittance to the University of Edinburgh medical school:

> "Miss Garrett and her strength!" writes S. J.-B. in her diary on May 19th, "making me break the 10th commandment. She doing Trigonometry, Optics, etc. Running where I crawl!"

They were not successful. Jex-Blake was still set on becoming a teacher, and resolved to study the best methods of education for women in Europe:

> Previously to this decision, S. J.-B. had published sensible letters on the subject in *The Scotsman*, *The Daily Review* and other papers. She also drafted an amusing letter in reply to her own, supposed to have been written by one of the retrogressive "unco guid."

> "Well, it was grand fun," she says in her diary, "and, if it had got in, might have played very well; but the chief temptation was the immense fun it would be. E. G. and I both thought we could command our faces.

> Her great desire for years had been to

fit herself for the work of a teacher, to found—or assist at the founding of—a wonderful college and (as the very height of her ambition) to be perhaps herself the headmistress. As she had planned Sackermena of old, so now she drafted detailed schemes of work, organization, finance.

She travelled to Germany and secured a position as a teacher:

Finally she applied for the post of English teacher in the Grand Ducal Institute at Mannheim.

As the Institution had embarked on a policy of strict retrenchment and economy, this was refused, but she had quite made up her mind to become an inmate in some capacity (as an ordinary pupil if necessary) and finally she set out without announcing her intention, in a fashion that recalls an adventure in the life of Lucy Snow in *Villette*. The condensed account of this in her diary could scarcely be bettered:

She enjoyed her work there, but encountered problems:

At work again! And, thank God, with such

strength for it! A new sap and strength in all my veins,—my heart in songs of gladness.

The heavy burden seems to have rolled away,—the sting and bitterness quite gone; strength and power returned to my hand,—colour and brightness to my life. Again I understand 'the thrill, the leap, the gladness'—again the sunshine has broken over earth. Now I go up and down the long corridors, catching with my hand at a great beam, in 'superfluous energy' again, (my darling!)—a smile over my whole face as I think I will tell her of my life in this weird old monastery—young bounding life all around—I myself no longer 'going softly'.

'Thank God! Thank God!' I can say nothing else."

How *can* people paint a teacher's life as always such a suffering one!

Eventually she tired of her work and decided to travel to the United States to study teaching methods there:

She poured out the story of her failure to her Mother, and delightful were the letters she got in reply:

"(Miss v. Palaus) will miss my darling and her unselfish love terribly when she leaves.... Without any great vanity you must know that your hearty ready help must be most refreshing to her, and your wide-awake state must have a great influence over the Girls."

In spite of all, however, the trouble went deep, and she chronicles sadly in her diary that "neither moon nor stars for many days appeared." Oddly enough, she never seems to have entertained the idea of simply giving in her resignation and going home. She entirely meant to serve her time,—nay more,—to hold the position until some suitable person was found to carry on her work.

She had a great scheme of going to America to study the education of girls there.

She traveled to Boston in 1865:

So she utilised every opportunity of getting information likely to help in her study of the conditions of Women's education. She regretted in after life that her dislike of 'lion-hunting' had prevented her from making—or cultivating—the acquaintance of well-known people who did not seem likely to be of direct help in her work. Not that she disdained the opportunities when they actually came within reach.

She was initially very impressed by the state of women's education in America:

I'm afraid that while we may have some few hundreds better educated,—more 'elegant scholars'—than any in America, we must confess that there is here a very much higher percentage of fairly well read and well educated people than with us. I notice this specially among the girls—as to the men I know less. But almost all girls here have studied a good deal things few English girls go much into—specially Mathematics and natural science.

Then I am sure no one ought to speak more highly than I of American kindness and hospitality,—I am very much afraid few foreigners would have found in England such a welcome as I met with here. People were so cordially kind in helping me in all sorts of ways.... There seems to me much less of the spirit of 'pride of office,' etc., much more readiness to admit one everywhere to see everything, and to be ready to help without standing too much on one's dignity.

"Sept. 9th. Went over to Concord, Mass. by 11 a.m. train. At the station found Waldo Emerson just fetching his wife and friends. I spoke to him and he very cordially asked us to 'take our dinner' with him.

Mr. Emerson struck me as having one of the sweetest expressions I have ever seen on a man's mouth. He was very kind in offering help.

She enjoyed the company of women doctors in Boston, and began to help out in a dispensary:

"You don't know," she writes to her Mother, "what an immense thing it is for us to have got free admission to the Woman's Hospital life here,—we are always doing something jolly together with the students and doctors,—all women, by the way.

She gradually became interested in medicine as a profession:

Darling, one very unexpected result is coming out of this new life which I embraced simply for its rest and comfort,—I find myself getting desperately in love with medicine as a science and as an art, to an extent I could not have believed possible. I always associated so much that is repulsive and nasty with it in my mind, but I find that one really loses all sense of that in close contact,—that the beauty of nature's arrangements and of art's contrivances absorb one's mind from everything less pleasant, and I find myself saying to myself a dozen times a day that, did I not feel my life devoted to another object, I would be a doctor straightway.

After two years in the U.S., her father became ill, and she returned to Britain. Soon afterward, he died:

In August, when S. J.-B. and Miss Heaton were abroad together, Miss Hill writes:

"London feels strangely desolate, the lamps looked as they used to look, pitiless and unending as I walked home last night, and knew I could not go to you.... I don't the least suppose you'll go to Florence or see my sisters, but, if you should, pray take off your 'spikes' and remember ... how much they love England, and everyone who is a friend of ours. I look forward to bright long days in which I shall learn always more about you, and watch with unending and unfathomable love and sympathy your upward growth, and we may look back together on our lives, as I do often on my own, and wonder how I could know and see so little, and wonder more how, knowing so little, I should be led continually to deeper truth."

Up to this point the friendship had been an almost unqualified gain, but, little by little, Miss Hill began to feel the strain of dividing herself—so to speak—between her family, her comrade and her work. In May 1861 she was called away by the illness of her friend, Miss Harris, and the change to an ideally peaceful life was just what she needed.

Jex-Blake returned to America, studied medicine in Boston and New York, and continued to ponder a career in medicine:

On September 1st, 1866, S. J.-B. sailed again for America. A warm welcome awaited her, and she speedily fell back into her niche at the Women's Hospital.

Having happily despatched her book, she was free to give her whole mind to the subject of Medicine, and she seems now to have enrolled formally as a medical student.

She saw that the need of adequate Graduation—urgent though it might be—was as nothing compared to the need of adequate Education. It *was* hard to make bricks without straw.

In April, 1867, the following correspondence was published in *The Boston Daily Advertiser*:

[Correspondence between Jex-Blake and Harvard University President regarding Jex-Blake's attempt to be admitted to Harvard Medical School. Her application is denied.]

A month later S.J.-B. had obtained introductions to each of the professors in the Medical Faculty at Harvard, and to each member of the staff of the Massachusetts General Hospital and of the Eye and Ear Infirmary: as well as to many people of standing connected with these various institutions: and she now proceeded to canvass them systematically. In addition to a number of influential friends, she was ably supported by Miss Dimock.

S. J.-B. quotes the above and a number of similar letters in the diary, and adds the comment:

"All which ends in ... smoke!"

Jex-Blake eventually returned to Britain and, after much consideration, determined to settle in Edinburgh and begin a medical practice.

Most Famous Quotes

Here are five of the most famous short quotations from *The Life of Sophia Jex-Blake*:

1. **"The breaker is gone up before them."** This quote, used to describe Jex-Blake's role in advancing women's education, signifies her pioneering spirit and how she paved the way for future generations.

2. **"It was *noblesse oblige* always,—the *noblesse* of family as much as the *noblesse* of Christ."** This quote reveals the complex social context in which Jex-Blake operated, acknowledging her family's aristocratic background and their commitment to social responsibility rooted in

their Christian faith.

3. **"Give a fair field and *try*'"** This concise statement encapsulates Jex-Blake's central argument for women's access to education and professional opportunities. It emphasizes her belief in women's capabilities and the need for equal opportunities to prove themselves.

4. **"Not me, but us."** This phrase became Jex-Blake's motto, highlighting her dedication to the collective advancement of women rather than individual success. It emphasizes her commitment to social change and her understanding that individual achievements were part of a larger movement.

5. **"'They also serve who only stand and wait';"** This quote from John Milton's sonnet "On His Blindness," underscores the difficult position of women who supported Jex-Blake's cause but were unable to participate actively. It also hints at the complex emotions of those who were forced to wait for societal change.

These quotes capture Jex-Blake's determination, her social context, her core arguments, her commitment to collective action, and the challenges faced by those who supported her cause.

Browsable Glossary

Perusing this glossary is cause for reflection on how readers a century ago routinely processed Latin and French terms that would be shielded from modern readers.–Ed.

A Visit to some American Schools and Colleges. The book that propelled Jex-Blake into public view, introducing her view of American educational methods to the British.

Alii. And others. [A common abbreviation for citing multiple sources.]

Annus mirabilis. Wonderful year. [1877 was a great year for women in England, but Jex-Blake lost her dearest friend. It was a year of triumph and loss.]

Arrière-pensée. A mental reservation; an ulterior motive.

Bene actæ vitæ recordatio jucundissima est. The remembrance of a well-spent life is most pleasant. [The words chosen by her son to appear on Sophia Jex-Blake's tombstone.]

Bene praeparatum pectus. A well-prepared heart. [The motto of the Jex-Blake family, chosen by some unknown ancestor. Did that ancestor know how profoundly it would fit Sophia?]

Bis dat qui cito dat. He gives twice who gives quickly. [Sophia took this to heart: she was always giving, and giving generously.]

Bonne bouche. A tasty morsel, a delicacy. [Father Duggan's dog liked to crunch a sugar cube at the end of tea time.]

Brocard. A legal maxim.

Caveat. A warning or proviso.

Ces jours heureux où nous étions si misérables. Those happy days when we were so miserable. [How many of us have looked back and said this. Even the happiest of lives contain some sorrows, and it's these sorrows that sometimes seem to bring the most delight when we recall them. And this is especially the case with the great sorrows. There is nothing so healing as time, time and change.]

Civis Academiae Edinensis. Citizen of the Edinburgh Academy. [This is what Jex-Blake became when she first matriculated at Edinburgh University, but many did not welcome the new citizen.]

Clientèle. Clients, customers.

Commune. A radical socialist government that ruled Paris in 1871.

Comte. Count. [A Comte is a Count in France, of course. And an Earl is a Count in England. And a Graf is a Count in Germany. And an Earl is also a Graf. There is no end to these aristocratic entanglements.]

Confrères. Colleagues.

Contretemps. A mishap, an awkward occurrence.

Corpus vile. A worthless thing. [Why should *this* University be the *corpus vile* for testing an unknown quantity? was a common refrain in those early days. And indeed it *is* asking a great deal of an institution to take the risk of alienating its supporters by trying a new experiment, especially if the experiment is not an obvious improvement, as was often the case when women asked to be included. Change for change's sake is not necessarily an advantage.]

Coup de mort. Death blow. [A love letter, inadvertently preserved, attests to this in a surprising context. And how much more might be said of that falling in love with medicine!]

Cri du Coeur. A cry from the heart.

Crux. The essential or deciding point.

Déjeuner. Lunch.

Déterrée. Disinterred.

Dévote. Devoted, devout, pious.

Défauts. Faults, shortcomings.

Dilettanti. Amateurs.

Dossier. A set of documents relating to a particular person or matter. [Sophia loved creating dossiers.]

Ébauche. A rough sketch, an outline.

Éclat. Brilliance, distinction.

Égalité. Equality.

Enfant gâtée. Spoiled child. [An apt designation for Sophia in her youth.]

En masse. All together.

Esprit d'escalier. Staircase wit; thinking of a clever retort too late.

Ex officio. By virtue of office.

Extra-Mural School. [Medical] classes conducted by lecturers who are not university professors.

Faux air. False appearance.

Fiat Voluntas Tua. Thy Will Be Done. [The unspoken watchword of Sophia Jex-Blake's life.]

Grande dame. Great lady.

Grossherzogliches Institut. Grand Ducal Institute.

Hadden down. Held down, kept down.

Hip Hip Hooray! A strange echo this from the old days of "Sackermena and her Isles," but now the warrior princess had grown to womanhood, and the child's game had taken on a real and serious import. "I do not know when I have felt so pleased and elated," wrote the recipient of this hearty greeting.

In limine. At the outset.

In statu quo. In the same state; unchanged.

Joie de vivre. Joy of living.

Jugement d'escalier. Staircase judgment; thinking of a better judgment too late.

Lachrymae rerum. Tears for things.

Lancet. A prominent British medical journal.

L.S.A. Licentiate of the Society of Apothecaries.

Magna pars. A great part.

Mailie'. A pet sheep at Surgeons' Hall. [The students had a sense of humor!]

Malice prepense. Malice aforethought.

Man-Midwife. A male doctor who delivered babies. [The very idea!]

Matin. A leading newspaper in Paris.

Métier. Profession, occupation, trade,

Minutiae. Trifling or insignificant details. [S. J.-B. was a master of detail. Her friends learned that, when she asked for a summary, it had better be precise!]

Modus Vivendi. Way of living; a practical compromise.

Nationalité. Nationality.

Noblesse Oblige. Privilege entails responsibility.

Nom de plume. Pen name.

Non tali auxilio, nec defensoribus istis. Not with such help, nor with such defenders. [A classic expression of dismay. One can imagine the feelings of the students when they read Dr. Bennet's letter to the *Lancet*. Their defenders—those of the orthodox school—were at times even more devastating than their adversaries.]

Par excellence. Preeminently. [Sophia excelled in

many ways. Her mother said she was an "excellent-natured" girl rather than a "sweet-tempered" one. Her fellow-students said she was an "out-of-the-way character." Sir James Stansfeld said that her mistakes actually helped the cause she fought for. And she herself said, many times, that she was "not strong enough for the place."]

Pari Passu. At an equal pace, side by side, together.

Partie Carrée. A party of four.

Per fas et nefas. By right or wrong.

Per omne fas et nefas. By every means, right or wrong.

Per persona. By hand.

Persona grata. A welcome or acceptable person.

Pluck. To fail an examination. [An amusing term, this. Evidently, chickens were not popular among examiners.]

Prex. Prayer.

Primâ facie. At first sight.

Propaganda. The spreading of ideas or information to help or injure a cause.

Protégée. A woman under the patronage or protection of another.

Qu'en pensez-vous?. What do you think?

Qui pauca considerat facile pronuntiat. He who considers little, decides easily. [Sophia, with all her impulsiveness, was not one of these. And she lost friends by this.]

Qui vivra verra. He who lives will see.

Quorum magna pars fui. In which I was a great part. [This was the opinion of Dr. Pechey's father, and he was no mean judge. "It is hard not to be envious sometimes," said Dr. Elizabeth Blackwell, "when one sees how generously Sophia has been appreciated." And she herself would have said that appreciation and friendship were all she cared for.]

Réchauffé. Warmed up. [A rehash, a warmed-over dish—how many of our thoughts and sayings are this! Sophia tried to avoid it. "Don't repeat the argument," she would say. "I remember all that."]

Reductio ad absurdum. Reduction to absurdity.

Régime. A system or course of living. [Jex-Blake was very fond of instituting regimes for her patients. She hated fuss and extravagance, but the proper food at the proper time was a cardinal point.]

Res merae facultatis. A thing of mere choice or possibility.

Résumé. A summary.

Rex. King.

Scotsman. A prominent Edinburgh newspaper.

Senatus Academicus. Academic Senate, consisting of the university professors.

Septem contra Edinam. Seven against Edinburgh. [The name by which the first seven Edinburgh students were known. And how gallantly they fought that losing fight!]

Se sauvaient. Saved themselves, ran away.

Sine qua non. An indispensable thing.

Soit. So be it.

Solvitur ambulando. It is solved by walking. [How different this from the solution that came by fighting and tears, and from the solution that came by the gradual evolution of mankind. It is not a question of merit. *Dis aliter visum.*]

Status quo. The existing state of affairs.

Summons. A legal document calling someone to court.

Sybarite. A person devoted to luxury.

Tapis. On the agenda.

Terrain. Ground, field. [As Professor Sidgwick would have said, "*Our* terrain is a slippery one."]

Times. A prominent British newspaper.

Trades-unionist. A member of an organization of workers, formed to protect their rights and interests. [Jex-Blake never had much sympathy with these. "The workers ought to get their rights," she would say, "but not by limiting work to incompetent people."]

Ultra vires. Beyond its power. [This was the decision of the Court of Session regarding the University of Edinburgh's attempt to graduate women medical students. What wonder if the University said, "We told you so." And what wonder, on the other hand, if the women students retorted, "Why did you admit us, if you didn't know what your powers were?"]

Une déterrée. Disinterred.

Verb. sap. A word to the wise is enough. [The newspapers of the period did not hesitate to apply this when a woman distinguished herself anywhere. If only it had had more effect!]

Vis-à-vis. Face to face with.

Vor den Wissenden sich stellen. To present yourself before those who know. [An admirable motto, but easier to carry out when youth and energy are one's supporters.]

Wee bit thing. A small thing.

Zeitgeist. Spirit of the times. [What the Zeitgeist was at the moment when Sophia Jex-Blake came to womanhood, we have only to glance at the foregoing pages in order to realize.]

Timeline

1840: Sophia Jex-Blake is born in Hastings, England.

1850: Jex-Blake takes a family trip to the Lake District.

1857: Jex-Blake leaves school and lives at home, writing stories and engaging in charitable activities.

1858: Jex-Blake begins attending Queen's College in London.

1860: Jex-Blake forms a close friendship with Octavia Hill, and they live together briefly.

1862: Jex-Blake travels to Edinburgh to investigate the possibility of further education there.

1865: Jex-Blake travels to the United States to observe women's colleges.

1866: Jex-Blake returns to America, intending to study medicine.

1867: Jex-Blake applies to Harvard Medical School, but her application is rejected. She begins studying medicine privately and working at the New England Hospital for Women and Children.

1868: Jex-Blake moves to New York, continues medical studies, and helps found a medical school for women. Her father dies, and she returns to England permanently.

1869: Jex-Blake and six other women matriculate at Edinburgh University.

1870: Miss Pechey is denied a Hope Scholarship. The women students experience increasing hostility from male students, culminating in a riot at Surgeons' Hall. The women begin a campaign to gain admittance to the Royal Infirmary.

1871: Jex-Blake makes an impassioned speech at an Infirmary meeting, which leads to a libel suit against her by Professor Christison's assistant. She wins the case, but is ordered to pay court costs.

1872: Jex-Blake publishes *Medical Women*. The University Court of Edinburgh refuses to make further provisions for the women students. The women bring an Action of Declarator against the University to compel the provision of complete medical education for women, including graduation. Lord Gifford rules in favor of the women.

1873: The University appeals Lord Gifford's ruling. Jex-Blake delivers a public lecture in London about her experience in Edinburgh. The Inner House of the Court of Session overturns Lord Gifford's ruling, and the women students lose their case.

1874: Cowper-Temple introduces an Enabling Bill in Parliament, but it fails to pass.

1876: The women students apply to the Royal College of Surgeons to sit for the License in Midwifery exam. After initially agreeing to accept the women, the examiners resign. The Russell Gurney Enabling Act passes, allowing all medical examining bodies to examine women.

1877: The Royal Free Hospital in London opens its doors to women. Jex-Blake graduates from the University of Berne and obtains the Licence of the Irish College of Physicians. She and Miss Pechey become the fifth and sixth women on the British Medical Register. Jex-Blake's mother dies.

1878: Jex-Blake settles in Edinburgh, begins a medical practice, and establishes a Dispensary.

1886: Jex-Blake establishes a small hospital in connection with her Dispensary, the nucleus of what would become the Edinburgh Hospital for Women and Children. She publishes a second edition of *Medical Women.* She delivers a free public lecture on women's health in Edinburgh. She is appointed lecturer on Midwifery in the Edinburgh Extra-Mural School.

1888: Jex-Blake establishes a separate School of Medicine for Women in Edinburgh.

1894: After a 25-year fight, the University of Edinburgh opens its medical school to women.

1899: Jex-Blake retires from Edinburgh and settles at Windydene, near Mark Cross, Sussex.

1912: Jex-Blake dies.

www.ingramcontent.com/pod-product-compliance
Lightning Source LLC
Chambersburg PA
CBHW060047050426
42448CB00012B/3145